The Fun We Had

A therapist in recovery writes about
addiction, poetry and the 12 Steps

CHRISTOPHER BURN

First published in 2016
by DHH Publishing
The Old Joiners Shop
Skirling by Biggar, South Lanarkshire,
ML12 6HD
Scotland, UK

Cover design by Christopher Burn and Manuela Boghian

A CIP record for this book is available from the British Library
ISBN 978-0-9934663-5-9

Also published by the same author:
Poetry Changes Lives: Daily Thoughts on Poetry and History

"You are never welcome in my life again. I already know what you're going to say because I've heard it before: 'what about the fun we had together?'"
From an alcoholic's goodbye letter to addiction

'The Fun We Had' is not euphoric recall, but the Siren Call of our addiction that never ceases.

DEDICATION

For all those involved in any way in the struggle
against addiction.
It can be beaten.

CONTENTS

ACKNOWLEDGMENTS

My thanks to Manuela Boghian and Rupert Wolfe Murray and my colleagues at Castle Craig Hospital, Scotland, for helping to make this book possible.

CHRISTOPHER BURN

FOREWORD

This book is a collection of articles and poems written over the past three years. Many of these items have appeared on the website of Castle Craig Hospital and the websites Poetry Changes Lives and Poetry Therapy News.

Addiction treatment is a serious business where pain often comes before gain and encouragement can make a huge difference; recovery on the other hand, should be enjoyed – it is the chance of a second life that should be taken wholeheartedly. Many recovering addicts find themselves doing and relishing activities that they never dreamt of before. They find themselves to be 'better than well'.

The Twelve Step Programme of recovery is unique in that it introduces the idea of spirituality, an idea formulated by Psychologist Carl Jung when writing to Bill W (co-founder of AA) in 1934 as 'spiritus contra spiritum' (ie: spirituality against alcoholic spirits). Spirituality is usually profoundly lacking in those in active addiction but the process of enquiry into this, in recovery, is for many a fascinating and life changing experience.

I hope that this book will provide some insights into both addiction and the enjoyment of recovery.

INTRODUCTION

Chaos and catastrophe were our lifestyle choices. Accepting the unacceptable our default attitude. 'Oh f***, I've done it again' our waking thought. No wonder we got happy when it all stopped – miracles do that to you.

The lunatic in the asylum who stops beating his head with a hammer is deliriously joyful. After thirty years of self-destructive behaviour, I know exactly how that feels.

I have a deep fellowship with that lunatic, because I am one myself.

I will always be a lunatic and I know how to find that hammer, if I choose to. I am an addict and I will always be an addict but miraculously, I am now a happy addict.

How did that happen? I have absolutely no idea.

It certainly involved a process of change and acceptance; it needed help from others – their example, experience and empathy; it required converting pride, dishonesty and ego into humility, honesty and unselfishness; it included some education and listening; but the fact that it actually happened, rather than being just a concept of how change might one day occur, is why it is a miracle. And miracles come from God – a God of our understanding, perhaps an Unknown God in many senses, but crucially, a Power Greater than Ourselves.

But it does not stop there. By opening our minds in this way, spirituality shows us a brilliant new life where anything is possible and hope, love and gratitude are there to be explored. Discovering this is like awakening from a nightmare, like being reborn.

American beat generation poet Allen Ginsberg used a lot of drugs in his life. This poem of his says it all to me:

I never dreamed the sea so deep,
The earth so dark; so long my sleep.
I have become another child.
I wake to see the world go wild.

The 12 Step Programme pioneered by Alcoholics Anonymous is highly effective and unique in that it introduces the idea of spirituality into recovery from addiction. By doing so, it takes us away from our self-obsession and selfishness; we realise not only that we aren't alone in our struggles, but also that help is available. It is a journey of discovery that saved my life, and for that I am grateful to it.

This small book covers some points on the journey from 'terminally unwell' to 'better than well'. You don't have to be an addict to read it but if you're not – this is what you're missing.

THE FALL INTO ADDICTION

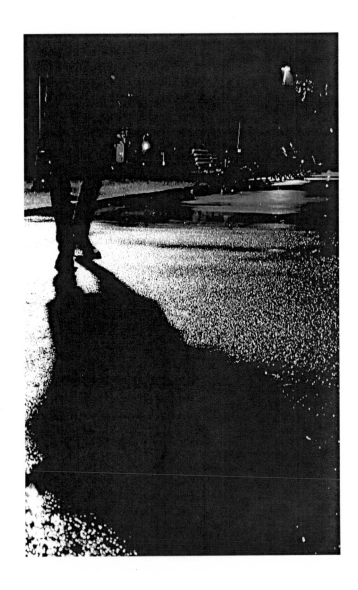

A Shadow

Indistinct to human eyes
Shadow on the pavement lies.
Gliding over stones at will,
Never hasty never still.
Memory of darker days –
Nights engulfed in amber haze.
Fearful of a world too wild –
Symbol of the inner child.
Always careful not to show
Secrets you must never know.
Quick to judge but full of fear –
You're too far and I'm too near.
Full of anger full of shame,
Always passing on the blame.
Everything begins with me –
Hiding from reality.
This is how the past was made,
Followed, followed by this shade.
A shadow on the pavement lies –
Box it up and tie the ties.
Place it safely on the shelf –
Shadow of my former self.

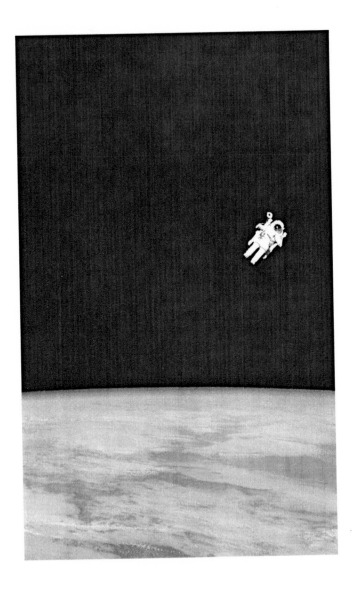

Spaced Travel

In 1958, an episode of the BBC's legendary Goon Show featured a trip to the moon by its characters, Seagoon, Bloodnok and the rest. The somewhat unlikely vehicle for the trip was the Albert Memorial, Queen Victoria's magnificently ornate tribute to her beloved consort – usefully pointy but probably not airworthy, let alone space-worthy. In 1958 the odds against a moon landing in the near future were probably several thousand to one. So did Professor Seagoon and the resourceful Major Bloodnok make it to the moon? I doubt it. In fact, when I checked it out last week, the Albert Memorial was still firmly anchored in its usual place in Hyde Park, opposite the Albert Hall. Spike Milligan, scriptwriter extraordinaire and main creator of the Goon Show, was famously bipolar and, reportedly, alcoholic. His flights of fancy were often beyond bizarre and took him to many strange worlds.

In 1958 I was a teenage space cadet and had already been to the moon many times, mostly to the dark side. My rocket fuel was a mixture – a spliff would give lift-off, whisky for the long haul and a few pills for touchdown. It was pretty dark up there alright. That was where things were done differently; where nothing was real, where people were just faces, where actions were simply reactions, where the past was a crater-strewn plateau of failures and the future an opaque mountain range of anxiety. In such a country, the only currency is illusion – reality is just too painful to use. Indeed, what is the point of reality when you are not capable of taking sensible action? Better to stay in wonderland, in the Xanaduian dreams of the addict where anything is possible and nothing is do-able; where unrealistic thinking is the norm.

So what has changed since then? Well, a Saturn rocket twice the height of the Albert Memorial, put a real man on the moon in 1969 – a triumph of technology, project management and joined up thinking that Major Bloodnok no doubt would have admired. As for my own space travel, perhaps I have been learning what true reality is and how the earth-people deal with it; how to achieve my needs rather than my desires; how to dream, but make my dreams achievable; how to be responsible for my own life. For me today – I am still a traveller but perhaps more a star sailor than a space cadet – I can navigate and I have a destination. We are in a joined up universe but we live on earth. In the words of the Goons again:

Seagoon (trying to explain gravity to Eccles):

'Jump in the air … So, why did you come back down?'
Eccles: 'Well, I live 'ere'.

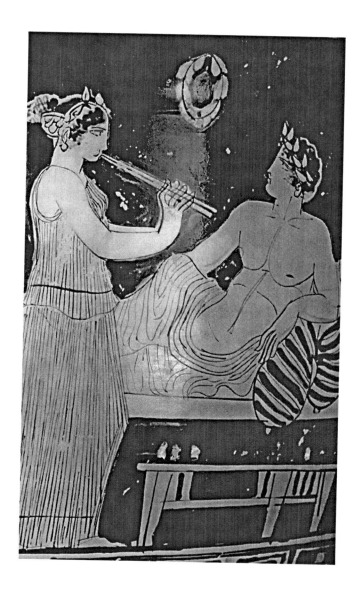

Ancient Addictions

Was Alexander the Great an alcoholic? Did Odysseus take opium in the land of the lotus-eaters? Was the romance of Anthony and Cleopatra an alcohol fuelled orgy, and was the Oracle at Delphi the world's first rehab?

Hold on a minute, wasn't the classical world of ancient Greece and Rome supposed to have been a truly blessed place where human behaviour and its consequences were perhaps for the first time, studied and understood; where people tried to live up to superhuman ideals and where (in literature at any rate), gods interacted physically with humans? In this materially simple but intellectually sophisticated age, weren't men and women supposed to have lived lives according to both man made laws and divine guidance, that gave them moral, spiritual and ethical values that are the envy of the world today? The plays of Sophocles and Euripides are full of this sort of thing. Doesn't all that add up to a truly golden age? Nobody ever mentioned addiction or character defects among the heroic men of that time, when we were at school, did they? Yet as so often with history, the facts are sometimes ambiguous and open to interpretation.

Alcohol was widely accepted then as it is today and cannabis and opium were certainly known , though not generally used, so presumably there must have been some sort of addiction problem too. There always is.

Take that famous institution of the Greek world – the Oracle at Delphi; people came to this place (the temple of Apollo) at points of crisis in their lives, to help them make decisions and to ask for advice. Significantly, the temple was also one of the most important sites for the cult of Dionysus, god of wine and the regulation of the Bacchanal ceremonies associated with the cult, involving heavy drinking and orgies. Written on the walls of the temple itself were many pithy phrases that echo down the ages to resonate with addicts today. For example: 'water is best', 'know thyself', and 'nothing in excess'. Several utterances survive of the oracle itself; many are political in nature but fragments such as 'the strength of lions or bulls shall not hold him, for he has the power of Zeus and will not be checked' ,point to an emphatic religious belief. The Greeks were very aware of the dangers of over indulgence in alcohol, their literature alludes to it often. For example, the Roman historian Seneca wrote that 'excessive alcohol will destroy the mind and magnify character defects' (his words, not mine) .

How tantalising it is to wonder if the oracle at Delphi, with its control of the cult of Dionysus, god of wine, its recovery – jargon slogans and its spiritual utterances, might perhaps have offered an alcohol counselling service as well as its other functions. Could it be that we are looking at the world's first rehab? Were these the early ideas that lie behind today's well used twelve step programmes: look again at those Delphic quotes: 'water is best' (step one?), 'the power of Zeus' (step two and three?), 'know thyself' (step four?).

If recovery was going on at Delphi, there would have been plenty of customers; top of the A list celebrities being Alexander the Great of Macedon. He is on record as having publicly insulted his mother in law at a drunken banquet, killing his close friend Kleitos in the course of another drunken banquet and finally setting fire to the royal palace at Persepolis, a city he had just conquered, in the course of yet another drunken banquet! Whatever treatment he might have had seems to have failed however, because his death at an early age from a mysterious illness, bears some of the hallmarks of alcohol dependence.

Then there is Marcus Antonius of Rome, famous as Cleopatra's other half, of noble birth but with a reputation for heavy drinking and a known gambling problem. As the historian Seneca put it: 'What else was it but drinking to excess together with a passion for Cleopatra, that ruined that great and gifted man?' Certainly Mark Antony's foray into Egypt which began well, descended into chaos and disaster in a way that will seem familiar to a lot of addicted people today.

Amusing true stories also survive about ordinary people getting drunk like the one recounted by the historian Athenaeus. He explains why a certain house is called 'the trireme' (a ship). It seems that some young men living there got drunk and thought they were at sea, sailing in a trireme. Encountering (they thought) a bad storm and fearing that the trireme might sink, they began to lighten the load by throwing furniture out of the upstairs windows of the house. The magistrates came to investigate the uproar and some arrests were made – clearly heavy intoxication took place in 'the trireme', of the kind you might easily find in any city today.

Lastly, though perhaps he should have been first, we come to Homer, whose amazing works were probably written or put together by several people, about three thousand years ago. In the Odyssey (the journey of Odysseus home from the Trojan war), we have several instances of both drunkenness and drug taking. In one example, Odysseus plies the one – eyed Cyclops, Polyphemus with strong wine until he passes out then blinds his eye with a sharp stick (thus making him history's first blind drunk). In another episode, Odysseus' ship arrives at the land of the lotus eaters and the crew get zonked out eating a plant that certainly wasn't a lotus – it was probably opium or cannabis, of which both are recorded as available in classical times though their use seems to have been limited.

So what, you might be tempted to ask, is the point of all this? Well, we have, I think, established that in the classical world, the use of alcohol was widespread and excessive drinking happened quite often. In addition, drugs such as opium and cannabis were certainly known and available, though not widely used. The big unanswered question is this: if alcohol was widely used in the ancient world and if some other drugs were also available, was serious addiction a problem and if so, how was it treated? Again, were there alcohol and drug dependent people wandering the streets of Athens and Rome, and what happened to them? Did any recover? We will probably never know. Perhaps the answer lies buried at Delphi.

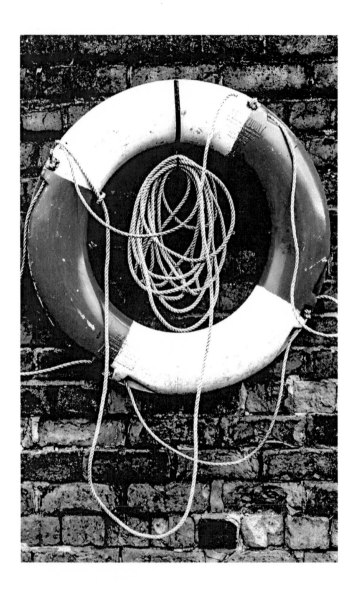

Are You Enabling Addiction?

Where there is addiction, there is usually enabling by those close to the addicted person.

What is enabling?

It is shielding the addicted person from the natural consequences of their addictive behaviour. Examples of this might be: giving them money to buy drugs or pay off debts: fulfilling commitments that the addicted person cannot honour; or even bailing them out of jail. It happens a lot and it is usually the result of strong and confused feelings (fear, guilt, anger, and despair) that loved ones have towards the addicted person in their midst.

Enabling behaviour often starts through a well – intentioned desire to help, but can quickly turn into crisis management and desperation.

Fear of the consequences of not enabling can be huge: for example, a wife might cover up for a husband not attending his work, for fear of him losing his job. (But losing a job is in fact where reality starts for many and can be a big incentive to seeking recovery).

Often there is a difficult choice to make, when deciding whether or not to enable, between short term pain and long term misery.

Anyone who has lived closely with an addicted person should consider the word codependence. If you spend the day worrying about what your addicted husband will be like when he comes home and how you will react, if you feel that you can only be happy when they (the addict) are happy and if you are driven to rage at their behaviour, monitoring their intake and cleaning up after them every day, then you are most probably codependent.

You end up simply reacting to another's moods and actions. It is no way to live.

Families often do not realise that codependency is happening and how their enabling behaviour is developing.

Some family members may even be content to take on an enabling role – as nursemaid or protector, because it gives them the feeling of being needed.

Codependent people are basically sacrificing themselves to the needs of others, taking responsibility for their problems. A vital step in the recovery process is for family members and loved ones to recognise what is happening – that addiction is a family disease and that they have all in some way been affected by it. From that it follows that they will need to make some form of recovery themselves, just like the addict, because they may be as sick as them or even sicker.

Many families benefit by going to Alanon, the 12 step fellowship for families of addicts, where they can learn from the examples of others and receive support. Other loved ones get special counselling to help them.

One thing is for sure, a process of change will need to happen for most families or others who are close to the addict. It's called 'tough love'.

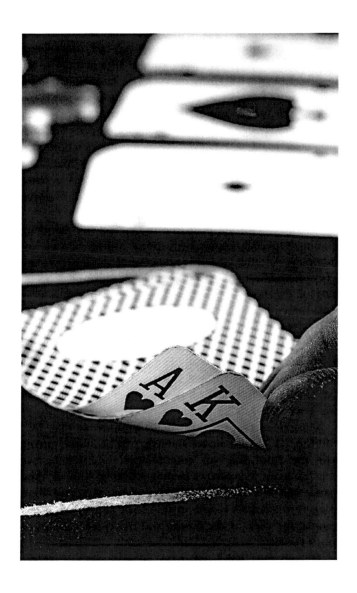

Behavioural Addiction – A 21st Century Threat

Diseases come and go and epidemics are often linked to trends in human behaviour. In the 19th century it was syphilis and other sexually transmitted diseases, while the 20th century brought us addiction to mood altering drugs and AIDS. What was not foreseen was that the 21st century would give us so much addiction directly linked to behaviour itself; in other words, as far as addiction goes, we seem to be gradually moving away from the 'highs' that come from the ingestion of chemicals towards a purer, though perhaps more dangerous, fixation with a virtual world which is now so readily available to us.

Examples of such addictive behaviours are gambling, gaming (especially mmorpgs), pornography viewing and shopping. Another emerging addiction is social networking where people can spend many hours a day fixated on the likes of Facebook or Twitter. It is no surprise that all of these activities can be done, though not exclusively, in the home. The provider of these behaviours is the computer which is linked to the Internet. In this way, Joe Public's home is not only his castle but has become his virtual brothel, casino, department store and battlefield where he can spend, gamble, campaign and pillage, worldwide, and 24/7, according to his tastes.

Illusions perhaps create other illusions. It may be a comfort for Joe Public to think that he is simply moving with the times, that any communication cannot be bad, that his brain is getting a healthy workout with all those games and that there is something a bit backward about going into a real shop with cash in hand and talking to real people; the click of the mouse and the credit card are so much cooler.

But, in fact, there are many adverse consequences – there always are with addictions. Leave aside the likelihood that regular long hours immobile in front of a screen are likely to make you overweight, the real damage is social and psychological. Isolation, loss of friends, family breakdown and financial disaster are common. Depression and even suicide are not uncommon.

Hospitals and clinics are already treating increasing numbers of behavioural addicts. Here at Castle Craig , the "Gambling and Compulsive Behaviours" Course is divided roughly three to one between gamblers and other compulsions, mainly gaming.

Although the American Psychiatric Association (who produce the diagnostic bible known as the DSM IV, soon to be DSM V) have not yet recognised many compulsive behaviours as addictive diseases, they are certainly moving that way and will in their next update (DSM V) classify compulsive gambling as such. As most other compulsive behaviours follow the same classic diagnostic criteria (tolerance, withdrawals, obsession, inability to control, loss of other interests, dishonesty, return to behaviour persistently), no doubt their classification will come soon.

Nobody really knows the extent of this behavioural addiction problem, perhaps it is too early to get reliable statistics. However, taking just gambling and gaming together, one could estimate that at least twenty million people in the UK do one or the other regularly. Assuming that 5% of them have a serious problem, one may say that at least one million people in the UK have a serious behavioural addiction.

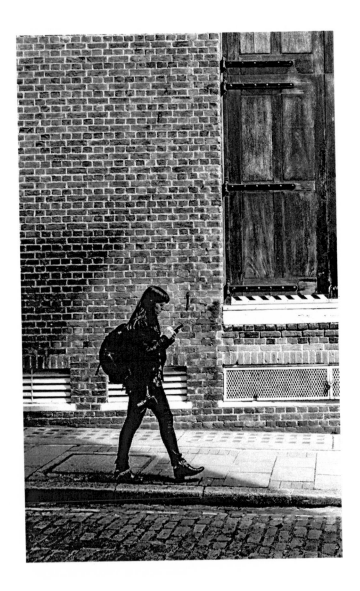

Text 'A' for Addiction

Beep Beep Beep...

It really is time to face up to another addiction that nearly all of us have, though nearly all of us minimise.

Can phone use be an addiction? Well the behaviour of mobile phone users certainly looks addictive; from a distance, phone use looks a bit like cigarette use except that people put phones to their ears instead of to their mouths. There is that look of gratification, of a need being met and an anxiety allayed.

So, are there serious consequences involved? Leaving aside the thought that all those little microwaves might be frying your brain every time you make a call (nobody seems too sure about that one), there are other possible consequences such as time wasted, undue dependence on meaningless communication, unrealistic thinking and expectations, money spent, loss of privacy and other interests.

And there are the consequences for society in general. Look at a movie from say 15 years ago, as I did the other day. I was struck by the easy way people moved – no measured pacing up and down, no one sided loud conversations in public places, no frantic scrabbling in bags and pockets to trace the ubiquitous beep. Why, I found myself asking, did we saddle ourselves with this electronic gadfly? Why did we choose to make ourselves answerable, textable, traceable, just plain available, 24/7? If a government had tried to impose such an idea upon us fifty years ago, there would have been uproar. We chose this ourselves and now it seems, we can't do without it!

Withdrawal, as any doctor will tell you, is one of the classic criteria for diagnosing addiction. Try living for a few days without your mobile and see how you feel – anxious, irritable, impatient, lonely, stressed, depressed, perhaps all at once – these are emotions commonly felt by most people.

Nomophobia, a word unknown five years ago, is the fear of being out of mobile phone communication. It is reckoned by some to be the fastest growing global phobia. Symptoms are constant checking of phones for messages and missed calls, inability to ever turn one's phone off, constantly topping up battery power, and taking one's phone everywhere, even into the bathroom. It is estimated that a great many of us, show some of the symptoms described above. Some people's lives can be made unbearable about this and there are already clinics where treatment is available. I suspect, however, that many of us shrink from taking this treatment because we fear that the cure will be worse than the disease.

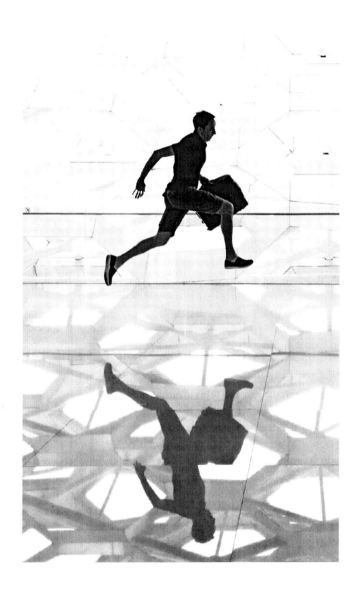

Is Workaholism an Addiction?

A recent article in the Daily Telegraph by Will Storr asked 'Are we a nation of workaholics?' and posed the question whether workaholism is a recognised addiction.

There is no generally accepted medical definition of workaholism. DSM IV (the Bible for diagnosis of mental illness) does not mention it. So, is workaholism an addiction? Some academics (such as Professor Robert West of University College London) are sceptical, saying that it is in human nature to indulge in compulsive behaviour in spite of the knowledge of severe negative consequences.

In Japan they see things differently. A nation of compulsive workers, they even have a word for death from overwork (karoshi). This was cited as the main cause of the fatal stroke of Prime Minister of Japan Keizō Obuchi, in the year 2000.

There have been WA (Workaholics Anonymous) meetings in Japan for several years but in general, karoshi in Japan is not viewed negatively.

One Japanese WA member is quoted as saying 'Karoshi is the modern version of seppuku (ritual suicide). It is considered an honour, the ultimate sacrifice.'

In the UK it is quite respectable to be a workaholic though the term is usually used jokingly. Indeed, there is a general assumption that to truly succeed in the workplace, you have to be a workaholic. Workaholism is often seen as a badge of honour. The UK media seem to encourage this idea too.

However, according to the Daily Telegraph, there is a growing Workaholics Anonymous movement and more and more people are presenting themselves at doctors' surgeries with symptoms of 'burnout'. Economic worries seem to increase the problem – a lot of people seem to think that they have a duty to work obsessively, despite the negative consequences for their relationships and health.

The past decade has seen an increased awareness of behavioural addictions with gambling, gaming, shopping and viewing porn being very much in the news. All these contain an element of escape from reality and there may be a part of this in workaholic behaviour too.

At its most extreme, workaholism can fulfil all the diagnostic criteria for a disease of addiction (the DSM IV cites: "preoccupation, increased tolerance, withdrawals, repeating the behaviour, adverse effect on lifestyle, negative effect on moral values and relapse"). For many people however, working excessively long hours to the detriment of health, home and happiness is simply business as usual and it should not be pathologised.

For most overworked and stressed – out people in the UK, what is needed is a re-evaluation of priorities so that a proper balance can be found in their lives. Some counselling may be helpful in this. Karoshi should not be an option.

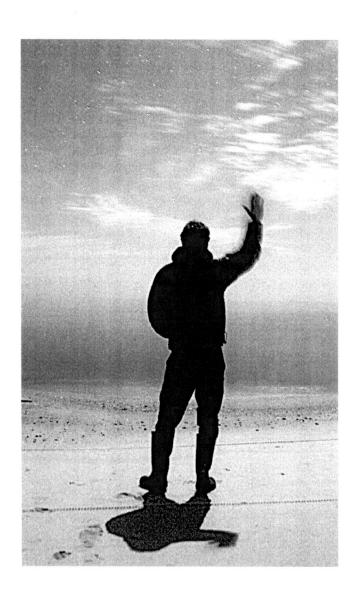

Goodbye Letter to Alcohol

A recovering addict wrote an anonymous "letter to alcohol" that I would like to share with you:

Dear Alcohol,
 a.k.a. tequila, gin, rum, beer, vodka, whisky, sake and any other aliases I may have missed
I am writing to say my final farewell to you once and for all.

We parted ways days ago when I walked out the door, hoping you wouldn't notice. You must have seen me leave because it wasn't long before you started begging me to come back. You promised that this time would be different.

You were right. This time it is different. It's no longer only me on the other end of the line. I've spent the last three months with many of your past loves, people who have broken up with you countless times. People who have learned to resist your charms.

They have taught me to do the same and I'm proud to say that I'm not coming back this time, choosing to forget all the pain and despair you've brought me over the past 30 years.

I know now how cunning, baffling and powerful you can be when you want to have your way with me. I've finally realized that I'm not as special as you said I was. You tried to convince me that I was the only one but the truth is there are many, just like me, whom you have left broken hearted.

You are never welcome in my life again. I already know what you 're going to say because I've heard it before: "What about the fun we had together?" Sure, there were good times, especially in the beginning when you were trying to make a good impression.

But those memories quickly faded as your true colours

began to come through. Your jovial mask came off and revealed the evil lurking beneath. I am no longer afraid of you because I'm no longer afraid of myself.

You only had power over me when I was powerless and unable to defend myself. You only prey on the weak and the vulnerable. You are a coward.

I will do everything in my power to expose you for the fraud that you are. I will join the others and help strengthen and support those unfortunate ones whom you've harmed with your lies and false promises.

We will continue to shine our light into your world of darkness until eventually it will simply cease to exist. I know that in the end love will prevail because it always does.

Goodbye and good riddance!

RISING FROM THE ASHES

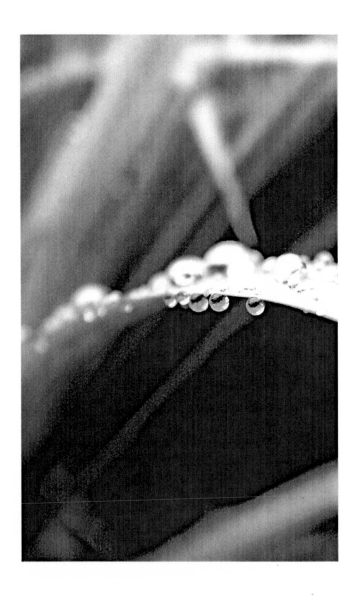

I Woke up Without a Hangover

I Woke up Without a Hangover
Shining, sparkling, spic-and-spangle
Daybreak-trance from dizzy dream –
Fluent, flowing, rushing,
Chasing
Spray - white horses through the green.
Sherbet fountains
Bubble - bursting
Rhythmic waves
And water-spouts
Erupting
Midst the bouncing stream.
Even I can tell –
That's better than well.

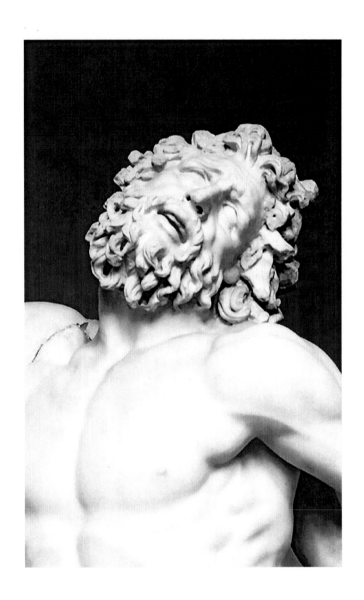

The Struggle of Addiction

For most of us there's something about the idea of change that we just don't like. Perhaps it's a fear of the unknown, or perhaps we just don't want to make the effort. However miserable we may feel, our current situation has become our comfort zone. Any change "might make matters worse".

Nevertheless, recovery from addiction is all about change. We have to change our old attitudes and practise new ways of doing things until they get so ingrained that they become new habits. Changing ourselves is a hard struggle.

But we know from working with thousands of cases that this kind of profound change is very possible. The keyword in the process is HOW: Honesty, Openness and Willingness to change. These are the three essential requirements for success.

Recovery from addiction is basically about regulating behaviour so that a new and better life can be built. The changes that have to be made during this process are difficult and take time. Later on we have to make sure these changes stay in place by diligently practising our new ways. Behaviour can normally only be successfully regulated if we make changes inside ourselves: to our attitudes, to the way we think and the way we respond to people and situations.

A person who is trying to recover from addiction, particularly in the early stages, is likely to be very occupied with the inner struggle between the new person they want to become and the old person that they are leaving behind. They may or may not be aware of this struggle, but it will be happening inside them and the symptoms will show themselves, including tiredness, irritability, anxiety and sleeplessness.

Addiction is a powerful, cunning and baffling disease

and it tries desperately to stay active within us. It will not give up or go away, in fact it will always be there waiting to attack us when we least suspect it. One of my patients used to liken addiction to Inspector Clouseau's sidekick Cato in the Pink Panther films .

The good news is that, as time goes by, this inner struggle will diminish in intensity. I believe that it will never go away completely, because addiction itself will never go away completely. We have a chronic disease and no matter how brilliant our recovery we will never receive a certificate telling us that we are cured.

The inner struggle never ends because there will, I believe, always remain a tiny part of us that does not want to change. And that tiny part is the remnant of our addiction – dormant and diminished but never dead. We forget this at our peril. We must never cease to regard recovery as work in progress.

Therapists working on "self-image" with a patient sometimes ask them to write an epitaph. The American poet Raymond Carver , a notorious alcoholic who was in recovery for the last seven years of his life, wrote this:

'And did you get what you wanted from this life, even so?

I did.

And what did you want?

To call myself beloved, to feel myself beloved on the earth.'

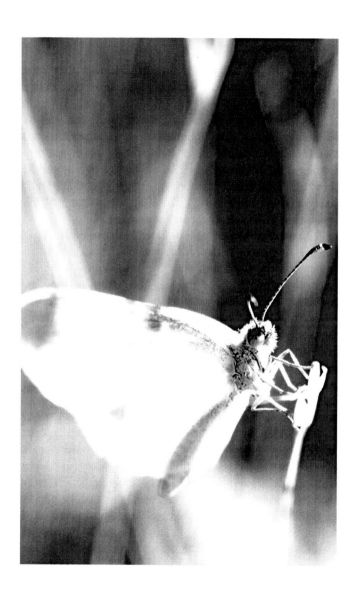

How People Change:
The Therapeutic Process in Recovery

Most people come to therapy because they want change to happen, and nowhere is this more true than in the field of addiction.

Addicts are often unrealistic; they expect someone else to change rather than themselves – a partner, boss or loved one. Sometimes they think that a purely external factor needs to change, such as moving to live in another country. Sometimes they even expect the therapist to change. They don't want to look at themselves; all they really want is a result: for the pain to cease.

The medical world has long been built around a passive 'doctor – patient' relationship, with the idea that the patient can lie back and wait for someone to fix them. Even the word 'patient' implies the act of waiting and enduring, rather than actively taking part in your own recovery. This is particularly problematic for addiction therapy, and newcomers to addiction treatment can have misconceptions about how it actually works. Often they think it will be like a hospital visit, that someone else is going to do all the hard work for them. But with therapy this is not the case. Nobody else can fix them. The patient has to take responsibility for this themselves.

Just understanding this fact is one of the hardest parts of recovery. Many addicts are stuck in 'victim mode', which means that they find it easier to blame circumstances or other people for their addiction rather than themselves. Blaming an unhappy childhood, for example, can be a perfect excuse for some to keep their habit going, while deciding to leave the comfort zone and do things differently can be a scary prospect. But it must be done. As the great psychotherapist and addiction expert Carl Jung said, "I am not what happened to me. I am what I choose to become" .

So therapy is all about change? Wrong – a large part of therapy is about acceptance. It is the combination of these two aspects that will make the therapeutic process work. As Reinhold Niebuhr put it in the Serenity Prayer :

"God grant me the serenity to accept the things I cannot change, courage to change the things I can and the wisdom to know the difference".

So how does therapy work in practice?

First off, the ground rules have to be established: at their simplest, the patient has to bring to the process the three basics of honesty, openness and willingness to change – without these, a successful outcome is unlikely. In return, the therapist must bring to the patient respect, empathy and understanding. With these ground rules in place, a healthy therapeutic relationship can be established.

But for progress to be made, it then becomes crucial for the patient to take responsibility for recovery, which means surrendering to the treatment programme and doing whatever it takes to recover, in the same way as a person with any form of terminal illness will follow a recovery programme that offers hope of success. In reality, these things are not so different: addiction too is often a terminal illness, if left untreated.

Then comes the often painful but essential process of facing reality, which will probably mean dealing with the denial that many addicts have towards their condition and its consequences. There are three essential truths that the patient must admit and accept:

- This is what your behaviour was like
- This is how it makes others feel and think about you
- This is how it makes you feel about yourself

By accepting this reality, the patient becomes ready to face the crucial questions: how do you feel about this situation and what do you, with help, want to do about it?

Getting to this point is hard, but there are two things that have proved incredibly effective in helping along the way: group therapy and something less tangible – the 'X Factor' of spirituality. Together, these two make up the corner stones of the highly unusual but remarkably effective model of the 12 steps program, which was introduced by the founding fathers of the Alcoholics Anonymous movement in the mid 1930's.

The inclusion of spirituality – the concept that recovering addicts need help from a 'power greater than themselves' (it does not have to be a God of any particular religion) – may be seen as a logical progression after the addict has fully admitted and accepted the powerlessness and unmanageability in their lives that was caused by addiction. By asking for help and exploring their spiritual side, many patients find that they are filling a void created by the absence of addiction.

It does not stop there however. In fact, it never stops at all, until we are dead. Change and acceptance can be undone and addiction is only ever in remission – an addict is never 'cured'. The new habits and attitudes that are learnt in the first periods of recovery must be nurtured even decades later. Sobriety can be the start of a happy and fulfilling life – but the price is eternal vigilance.

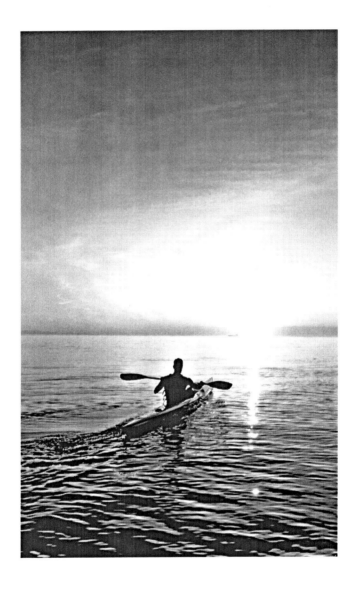

'Better than well' as a goal of treatment

The idea of 'better than well' in addiction recovery, has been around for a while. I guess people with addiction are never satisfied. When most people get over a sickness, they get back to 'normal' and carry on. Shouldn't 'well' be enough for addicts, after so much time being extremely 'unwell', or do recovering addicts have some secret that others don't have, are they dancing to a different tune?

Successful recovery from addiction represents a second chance. But real recovery is a very different thing to white knuckle abstinence.

When recovery is achieved through the framework of a 12-step programme, it goes far beyond the mere management of addiction. Through a process of self-discovery and change, the addict becomes a better and happier person with a zest for life that probably was not present even before addiction took hold.

In his book 'The Road Less Travelled' , the American psychiatrist Scott Peck talks of 'the blessing of alcoholism' by which he means that the crisis of alcoholism forces sufferers to address and improve themselves physically, mentally and spiritually and the twelve step fellowships are there to help them do so; those that join become better people – they become 'better than well'.

Recovery is a process. Such a transformation does not happen quickly and anyone in AA or NA will tell you that recovery never stops; it is a process. Various studies appear to show that something happens with addicts in their recovery, often at around the five-year mark. Before that point, many report feeling unwell, confirming the reality of early recovery as a struggle. But in marked contrast, once the first five years are passed, many acquire a greatly enhanced feeling of wellness which surpasses that experienced by the general public.

It is generally recognised that there are five ways to

achieving well-being or 'wellness':

- connect
- be active
- take notice
- keep learning
- give

All five can be found in a Twelve Step Programme and all one has to do is follow it. Wellness is often reported by those in recovery in the context of social activity and enjoyment of the environment. Visitors often express surprise at the enthusiasm and 'joie de vivre' that they see at fellowship meetings and conventions and ask 'what is their secret?' It calls to mind the words of Nietzsche: 'and those that were seen dancing were thought insane by those who could not hear the music'.

Many people in recovery consider themselves blessed indeed.

CHRISTOPHER BURN

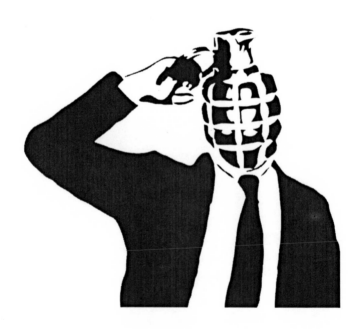

How to Sabotage Your Treatment

Most addicts like to wreck things. Throwing a spanner in the works when things are going well may be normal for some of us. Perhaps at one time it gave us an insane feeling of somehow being in control. Even in treatment we do this.

A twelve step programme requires rigorous honesty with self. This is a fundamental requirement. Compromise is not an option.

If addicts cut corners they start the process that leads to relapse.

Because addiction is so powerful and cunning, it will not leave us alone. It will try to get us out of treatment by playing on our weaknesses.

Consider the following list of 'sabotage thoughts':

1. I'm just out of detox and I feel better. I'll just go home because I know I can handle it now.
2. I can't really be an addict: I haven't lost my house, job, wife etc.
3. I don't want to deal with the here and now. It's too depressing.
4. My life has been so horrible it's no wonder I behave like this.
5. If you had my wife/father/boss, you'd be an addict too.
6. I'll keep doing things the way I always have, because I know best.
7. If I see someone with a problem similar to mine, I rescue them and don't let them deal with it.
8. I don't let my family come to family therapy – It'll save them emotional pain.
9. Drinking isn't a problem – I just want to control it.
10. I know the words 'one day at a time'. These are good words and I hope somebody puts them into action.
11. I know more than my therapist, especially about me.

12. I've learnt enough, I know about the steps and lots of things about AA/NA.
13. Look at John and Sue – they're really screwing up the programme.
14. I need to leave treatment. My boss needs me, my family needs me, my kids need me.
15. I need to hide my secrets. If I don't, you might not like me.
16. I don't need to work; my therapist is working hard enough for both of us.
17. These rules were made for other people, not me.
18. I don't like this place, the family will come and get me – after all, it's their responsibility.
19. If I want an intimate relationship with another patient it's our business and nobody else's.
20. I've learnt enough and I know I'll never use again – goodbye!

How can you deal with self-sabotage? As with all recovery, honesty is the keyword. Look at yourself, listen and ask for help. Remind yourself why you are in treatment and think of how it was before. Remember pride; it stops you listening to others, asking for help or relating to others. Learn to challenge your thoughts. Remind yourself again of what sabotage is: a misguided attempt to deal with negative thoughts by providing a quick solution. Don't let it happen.

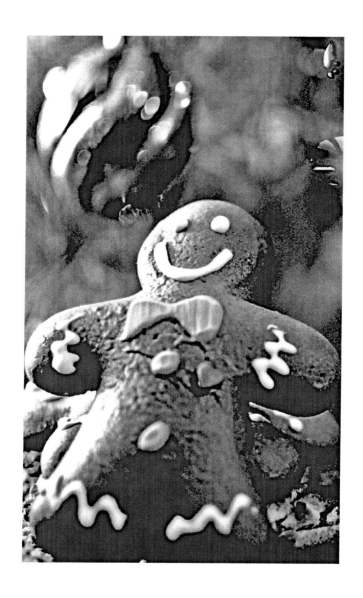

Christmas in Rehab

How do you view Christmas? As a time of happiness and inspiration, through its powerful symbolism of hope and salvation? As a time of anxiety, guilt and insecurity, derived from warped relationships and bitter memories? If you are in rehab or early recovery, then the latter is more likely. Like it or not, this once a year event can be a hugely disruptive influence that breaks up daily routine and plays havoc with our emotional balance.

Lots of addicts' view Christmas time with fear and loathing often for very personal reasons. But it does not have to be so. In rehab we are told that every situation is an opportunity – an opportunity to learn and to do things differently. So let's try and see it that way.

- Plan your days: Christmas can be a period when normal daily structures get suspended and there is more free time. So try to work out in advance how your day might go. Think about doing special things, perhaps helping colleagues who are needy. Plan to set aside time for meditation or prayer. We should be happy at Christmas, but don't expect a feeling of happiness to come without putting in some effort. Joseph Addison, the famous eighteenth century writer, once said: 'Three grand essentials to happiness in this life are: something to do, something to love, and something to hope for.' So try these suggestions:

- Give to others: not just presents (though that can be nice), but give your time, your affection and your talents, without expecting anything in return.

- Work on an attitude of gratitude: what is positive about my life, what can I be grateful for right now? Keeping a Gratitude Diary can help you focus on this and keep away negative thoughts.

- Think about goals for the coming year: what do you want to achieve, what would you like to be doing in a year's time? Christmas is a time of hope – we can all use a bit of that.

• Get in touch with family and loved ones: not to tell them how well you are doing but to ask how they are. Remember that all relationships seem to become doubly sensitive at this time – proceed with caution.

• View any social gatherings with care, especially if alcohol might be involved. Take prudent steps to ensure that you remain safe – go with an understanding friend or an escape plan if it all gets too much.

• Replace old self-defeating Christmas traditions (like wrapping presents while drinking a bottle of sparkling wine) with new positive traditions (e.g. going for a walk on Christmas morning).

• Keep an emotional balance; check yourself each day and if you're experiencing mood swings or unreasonable feelings of anger, loneliness, anxiety or depression, then do something about it – talk to someone, try to get to a fellowship meeting.

If you are feeling really negative about Christmas, try an exercise in challenging your beliefs:

• What negative thoughts do you have? For example: Christmas is a commercial sham; Christmas is an excuse for excess; Christmas is for fools; Nobody cares about me otherwise I'd be having a better time.

• Then ask yourself: what is the evidence for these beliefs and would a less dogmatic and less negative view be more helpful?

• What alternative thoughts would be more productive towards you having a good time? For example: There is a commercial side to Christmas but lots of people enjoy it without great expense. Some people overdo it at Christmas but I don't have to. A lot of very sensible people enjoy Christmas in a very meaningful way. I will have a better time if I don't isolate and make more effort to be sociable.

• Try discussing these points with other people.

Still feeling negative?

Negative thinking has been a habit for many of us and is part of the self-defeating cycle of negative thoughts, feelings and actions that probably ruled our lives for a long time. It won't go away easily.

Try this exercise: We all have memories of Christmases past, some good, some maybe not so good. How will you remember this Christmas? As a time when you felt lonely, unloved, insecure and inadequate? Or as the time when you finally decided that you did not have to live every day at the mercy of your emotions – that you could change your feelings by changing your thoughts, actions and attitudes? What do you actually have to do each day to make you remember this Christmas as a time when your hopes became real and you were re-born?

If you start taking positive action this Christmas, you will remember it as the moment when you began to change, as Ebenezer Scrooge did (in the book 'A Christmas Carol' by Charles Dickens) – I commend to you the final paragraph of that uplifting and enjoyable work:

'He (Scrooge) had no further intercourse with spirits, but lived upon The Total Abstinence Principle ever afterwards; and it was always said of him, that he knew how to keep Christmas well, if any man alive possessed the knowledge. May that be truly said of all of us!'

As an example of changing attitudes, 'A Christmas Carol' takes some beating. Why not read it this Christmas? I finish with its final words: 'And so, as Tiny Tim observed, God bless us, every one!'

LIFE AFTER REHAB

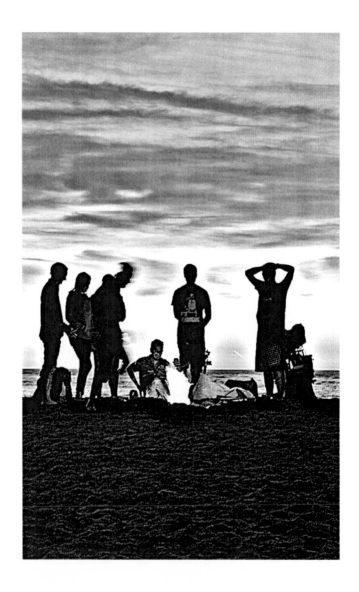

Fake it to make it, in AA

'Keep It Simple'. The words were written on a rather grubby looking card that was propped up on a shelf behind the speaker's table. Similar cards bore slogans like 'Easy Does It", 'A Day at a Time' and the enigmatic 'How Important is It?' The room we were in was cold and scruffy. I was not impressed. 'What', I asked myself again, 'am I doing in this place?'

In reality, AA was the last option. The runaway train that was my drinking career had finally hit the buffers. I had been there before as a sort of 'observer' (as I privately told myself). I didn't feel that I really needed it. The first meetings I'd been to had been boring and uncomfortable – all those people moaning about their drinking and pretending to be happy because they had stopped, were just phonies, it seemed to me.

It was only much later that I realised that, if you are in denial, any fellowship meeting is going to be uncomfortable. After all, if you have no intention of stopping yourself, why listen to a lot of people telling how they stopped?

An old chap called 'Lawyer Bob' put a paper cup of beige tea into my tremulous hand while a big bloke called 'Farmer Tom' said something loud and indecipherable while shaking my other hand. Other persons with weird names like 'Motorbike Willie', 'Sober Margaret', and the scary-sounding 'Meat Market George' came up and said hello. Such it seemed, was how anonymity was dealt with at AA. They were all cheerful and appeared to know and like each other very well.

That particular night, I was the newcomer and those sweet, kind people welcomed me unconditionally, as they always welcome newcomers. But on that night they didn't make me feel comfortable at all. I really didn't want to be there. Frankly, if I'd seen any of them getting on a bus, I would have waited for the next one. Such was my state of fear and denial at the time.

I stayed until the end of my first AA meeting because, deep down, I knew that I had to – I had no other options. The following week I went back again. And again. I still don't really know why.

Sometimes I was glad to go, sometimes I pretended to be glad to go. One time I heard an old timer say 'fake it to make it'.

Perhaps I was doing that. But some kind of miracle was happening because I wasn't drinking any more.

Twenty-eight years later, the room and the cards haven't changed at all. The welcome is just as warm and unconditional. Sober Margaret welcomes me with a kiss, Lawyer Bob and Farmer Tom are with their maker now, but there are others in their place. I know and love them all, they are my friends and my colleagues, my support and my guides and I have them to thank for my continued existence; it is their example, their love and their compassion that keep me sober. Today, I would be glad to see them at a bus stop and never even think of avoiding any one of them. There is a power in that scruffy room – a Higher Power.

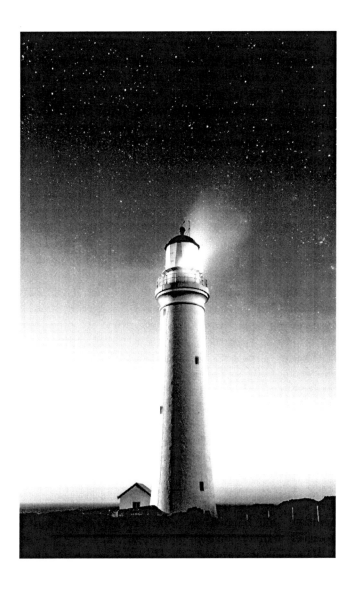

What is the Meaning of Higher Power?

The man who first nailed the idea of Higher Power was Professor Carl Jung. His famous play on words in a letter to AA co-founder Bill W, called it 'Spiritus contra Spiritum' – that is 'spirituality against spirits' (i.e. liquor). Like Jung, I find it impossible to talk about Higher Power without including spirituality. He compared the craving for alcohol with man's craving for wholeness with God, quoting the 42nd psalm: 'As the deer pants for streams of water so my soul pants for you, O God'.

All very neat, you might say, if you happen to be a Judaeo-Christian. Rather inconveniently, a lot of people in the 12 step fellowships are not Judaeo-Christian, are not religious or even god-believing. Clearly (as my Maths teacher used to say), there is more work to be done on this.

Perhaps we should start with the problem itself (that's how the 12 steps start): addiction is the problem and it destroys our lives – not completely, unless we allow it to, but one thing it always destroys is our spirit – this usually has more disastrous consequences than our actual misdeeds. Addiction turns us into emotional, moral and spiritual zombies. In the words of Oscar Wilde – 'it is not what one does that is wrong, but what one becomes as a consequence of it'.

This 'zombie' element in addiction has been identified by many in the recovery field as a key element for attention. One purpose in seeking a Higher Power in recovery, is therefore to get back for ourselves that spirit that we have lost through addiction; to re-connect with humanity and re-enter the joined-up universe. There is however, another aspect to the matter.

The main importance of a Higher Power is of course clearly stated in steps 2 and 3. It is about belief that help is available and asking for that help. Many addicts realise eventually that they need help and find it forthcoming from friends, fellowships or a variety of other sources. This is a good start. As reality dawns (if it does), they then accept that they are engaged in a life or death struggle with a deadly enemy, and they realise that they need some really powerful help if they are to come out winners. Fight force with force, get overwhelming power on your side.

If an Almighty God exists, then he is an absolute shoo-in for the Higher Power role, the ultimate Super power. It is really quite annoying that we can't prove for sure that he does exist. Plenty of us take the leap of faith, myself included, and are grateful for our beliefs. For the atheists and agnostics among us, it is not so easy. How can they, too, find a super power?

What can the person do who has no concept of God but has read chapter five of the AA Big Book and understands the need to find a higher power? Should he ignore it and carry on regardless? (not advisable), should he take Pascal's wager (there is a fifty-fifty chance that God exists so you might as well believe it and start praying – if he doesn't exist you lose nothing and if he does you win the jackpot)? should he 'fake it to make it'? (a possibility). I know many atheists in the fellowships and almost all have reached a point of finding a Higher Power that suits them, a 'God of their understanding', though the word 'God' may beside quite alien to them. They have managed this through following a process: accepting their own powerlessness, realising the need for help, understanding that only help that comes from a source of power will do, and then asking for that help. The actual help can take many forms, from their own fellowship group, to their sponsor, to a power for good throughout the world.

Agnostics too, abound in the fellowships. Such seekers after the truth generally have little problem, once they understand the principles behind steps 2 and 3. An open mind is the key. As the great seventeenth century thinker, Blaise Pascal put it, 'You would not seek God if you had not already found him'.

The 12step programme recognises the need for recovering addicts to find a Higher Power to fill the spiritual void, because they are powerless over their addiction and need help. This Higher Power can take many forms but it needs to be truly powerful.

Addicts in recovery have much to be grateful for. Through the 12 step programme they gain huge insights into themselves, their spirituality and their place in the universe. They learn to conquer their fears and live happily in sobriety with nothing in excess. The Delphic Oracle had some good points, but Higher Power is the key.

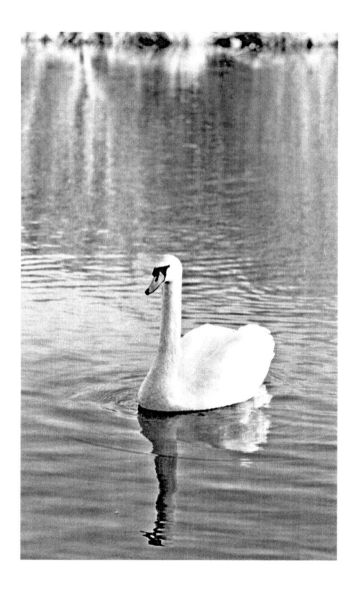

Ten Ways to Build Self-Respect

Most people who are recovering from addiction have a problem with self-respect. After all, if you have indulged in addictive behaviour that may have included lying, cheating, aggression and laziness, it is quite difficult to respect yourself.

The alcoholic who invents a 'business meeting' so he can spend more time in the pub instead of going home to his family, is acting against his conscience: he is lying, he is being selfish, he is causing distress to his family and he is spending his money in ways he should not. Deep down he knows this, his conscience tells him so, but he does it all the same and it makes him deeply unhappy – he will probably need another drink to help him cope with the bad feeling! Such behaviour, repeated regularly, cannot fail to erode self-respect.

Like happiness, self-respect cannot just happen upon you. It is important to understand this because many people, in desperate need of self-respect themselves, try quickly finding something to make them feel better: perhaps buying a new car or new clothes or displaying an arrogant behaviour in order to feel 'superior'. Or perhaps letting others invade their boundaries because any kind of attention makes them feel better.

Building self-respect in early recovery from addiction can be a slow but highly rewarding process. It combines elements of assertiveness, self-acceptance, spirituality, realism, focus, forgiveness, respect for others and humility. It is rewarding because you can see results and better still, you can feel them, as your self-respect increases. Try these self-respect building exercises:

1. Assertiveness: Recognise when people disrespect you and take steps to stop it. A person with self-respect doesn't allow others to treat them badly, and would rather not associate with someone who is disrespectful. When someone doesn't give you basic respect, you need to be able to say, in one way or another, "You just disrespected me and that's not acceptable."

2. Self-acceptance: Get to know yourself. The more you understand yourself, the more you'll appreciate how unique you are. Discover your own values, personality, and abilities. Stop people-pleasing and start developing your own character and standards. Be true to yourself. It is important you have faith in your own values and remember what is important to you. Just because other people think you should behave in a certain way, doesn't mean they are right.

3. Spirituality: True self-respect brings inner peace. Spirituality nurtures that inner peace. Do not reject this side of your personality. The journey towards spirituality can be an exciting and deeply satisfying experience.

4. Realism: Learn to handle criticism. We are sensitive beings. To maintain a sense of self respect, we need to learn how to deal with criticism. Don't take criticism personally. Look at it from a detached perspective.

5. Focus: It is motivation that matters, not actual results. The problem is that we equate our self-respect to outer displays of wealth, success and social standing – and this is a mistake.

6. Forgiveness: Forgive others and forgive yourself. Don't live in the past. Move on from past mistakes and difficult situations.

7. Respect others: If you have no respect for others, how can you respect yourself? It is the wrong approach to try to feel better by putting others down. If you look for good qualities in others, it will be easier to see the good qualities in yourself.

8. Humility: The way to self-respect is not through praise from others, which gives a false sense of pride. Be selfless.

9. Self-love: Never hate yourself. This can become a dangerous habit. We make mistakes, we may do the wrong thing, but we should never put ourselves down unnecessarily.

10. Responsibility: Make a conscious decision that you are no longer going to take the role of the 'victim' – you are responsible for your life and only you can make change happen. Joan Didion, an American author, says that "the willingness to accept responsibility for one's own life is the source from which self-respect springs."

Doing the above exercises and working on our self-respect means we are taking responsibility for our lives. We are no longer doormats, people-pleasers, self-deluders or self-haters. In short, we are ourselves – unique, independent, beautiful and self-respecting.

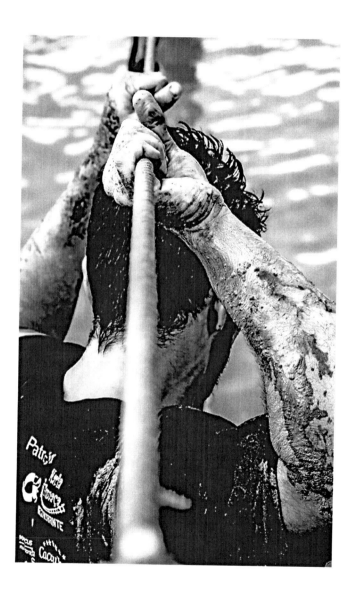

Coping with Cravings

In early recovery, just walking past a favourite bar or meeting a joint-smoking friend can be enough to start a strong craving; so can arguing with a family member or partner. Sitting in the sun and feeling really good can start cravings too. Or sitting in the rain! Help! Just about anything can start cravings! We'd better believe it. And we'd better be ready for them.

Addiction wants to return and cravings are a major method that it uses. When defences are weak and emotions still fluctuating, it is vital to be alert to the danger. Try to keep an emotional balance and remember HALT (don't be Hungry, Angry, Lonely or Tired).

Remember to take positive action. Do not be passive when a craving starts but have a plan in place that you can refer to. This should include the following:

- Remind yourself that cravings only last, on average, fifteen minutes.
- Do something immediately, however small. For example, a telephone call – a random number or the speaking clock even; you don't have to speak. Or clean your shoes, or your car. Do something.
- Relocate temporarily – go for a walk or call on a neighbour – it clears the mind.
- Speak to someone; arrange this person in advance, perhaps through the AA type fellowships.
- Use simple thought-changing techniques that you have already practiced such as counting the number of cigarette ends you can see (there are always some) or reciting a song or poem from memory.
- Rationalise and challenge your thoughts behind the craving: what is really happening here? Am I emotionally upset? Is this old behaviour returning? Am I just bored?

Action is crucial; never allow yourself to sit with the craving and hope that it will just go away. It won't.

Be very wary of impulsiveness when dealing with cravings. Many addicts are used to acting first and thinking later. A good way of combating this is to carry a Flashcard – a kind of visual wake-up call that can shake you back into the reality of your situation.

Such cards can be credit card size (keep them with your credit cards, payment is often a prelude to substance use) and might contain messages such as:

"Don't mess it up!"

A photograph of you in hospital after your last binge

Or "Don't be a ******!"

Longer term coping strategies will include learning mindfulness and meditation techniques, finding new interests, acquiring pets and house plants and even developing normal human interactions. By that time, the voice of the craving should be a lot smaller, but it may never go away completely.

Remember – cravings are just cravings – they won't kill you. In early sobriety, they can be very hard to overcome – taking the time to plan your response by learning some simple techniques, can make all the difference.

When cravings come, you must act. Doing nothing is not an option.

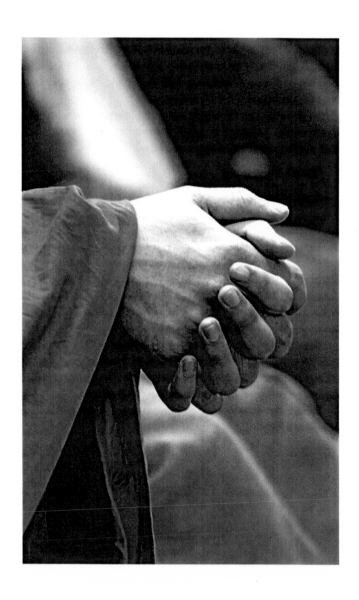

Non-verbal Communication

'I speak two languages, Body and English' (Mae West)

A least eighty per cent of communication is non-verbal, say the experts. You may raise your eyebrows at this statistic but it is certainly true. In fact, non-verbal communication often works better than the use of words. I am thinking of the expression of feelings: body gestures are far more effective to communicate the ideas of say, anger, sadness or anxiety, rather than simple verbal statements. Which has more effect on you, a person saying 'I am angry', or a scowling person invading your personal space with a red face and clenched fists? Probably the latter.

'The human body is the best picture of the human soul.'(Ludwig Wittgenstein)

While animals are highly effective in non-verbal communication, as anyone who has been chased by an angry dog will testify, it is probable that the human species managed quite well for thousands of years with just non-verbal communication, before language was introduced. In a simple world, language is not necessary, all you need to show are your feelings. For very small children the same is true. Language only becomes important as life becomes more complicated, when we need to give and understand instructions, exchange data and learn intricate techniques.

'The only language men ever speak perfectly is the one they learn in babyhood, when no one can teach them anything!' (Maria Montessori)

Today we find ourselves living in a highly complicated world: information has never been available in such quantity and the means of communication have never been so varied and so available. On the other hand, probably never have people misunderstood each other so much. This is partly due to the increasing trend of communication at a distance and the decline in face to face communication. Technologies such as Skype go some way to redressing this but the trend is still one that results in our gradual pulling away from regular meeting and intercommunication on a personal, physical level. As a result, we are becoming less skilled in 'reading' each other's non-verbal behaviour, so that our observations of people and what they are really trying to communicate, is on the decline.

'In the twenty first century there are too many messages and not enough communication.' (Anonymous)

We can probably all remember times when we have experienced failure in communication – this might have resulted from deliberate deception by another or from a genuine failure to read the signals. The consequences may not have been great but they could have been.

Perhaps as a teenager you (wrongly) failed to read the signs and thought that someone liked you a lot more than they in fact did – or perhaps the converse. If only you had been more skilful in reading the signs.

'There's language in her eye, her cheek, her lip, nay, her foot speaks; her wanton spirits look out at every joint and motive of her body.' (William Shakespeare)

If you get into the habit of checking another person's body language, and indeed your own too, you can learn a lot. Try looking at the following:

- Arms – folded (defensive), open wide (comforting),
- Hands – palms outward (fear), held to the face (surprise), fist (anger)
- Shoulders – shrugging (uncertain), drooping (sad), braced (powerful)
- Face – complexion (blushing), eyebrows (up – surprise), (down – aggression), nose wrinkling (dislike)

- Eyes – the mirror of the soul – eye contact is much more intent when we like another person, less when we dislike or are ambivalent. Consider also: winking, blinking, fluttering, rolling, narrowing.
- Legs and feet – shifting feet (insecurity), leg jigging when seated (impatience).
- Head – nodding (agreement), shaking (disagreement), drooping (defeat).

Non-verbal communication is a two-way street – not only can you observe others but you can communicate much more effectively yourself by employing your own body language.

As an exercise, you could try communicating with someone in a totally non-verbal way, and see if you can get your point across. Just consider smiling for example – how much power can be wielded in that simple act of non-verbal communication. The more you develop your non-verbal skills the better your contact with others will become.

'All you have to do is to pay attention; lessons always arrive when you are ready, and if you can read the signs, you will learn everything you need to know in order to take the next step.' (Paulo Coelho)

In therapeutic treatment, understanding non-verbal communication can be very helpful. In a group setting for example, probably everyone is sending out non-verbal messages of some kind; one person may be yawning (I'm trying to control the group), another jigging their foot (impatience) and a third may be pretending to sleep (get me out of here) while a person in denial may be showing signs of defensiveness (crossed arms). Try some conscious non-verbal communication yourself. Could you, for example, spend a whole day without speaking, just communicating non-verbally? It has been tried.

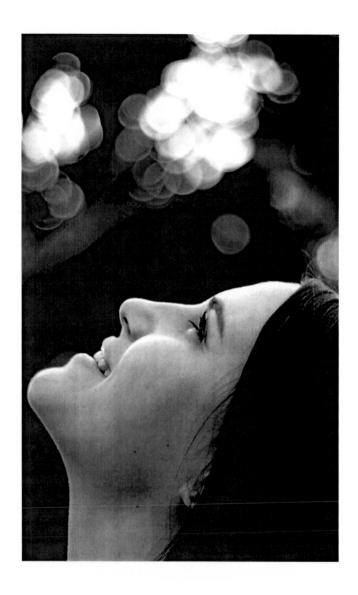

Are Women More Emotional than Men?

Men often complain that women are too emotional; women often complain that men are not emotional enough. These are stereotypes. Modern brain research is opening up factual evidence to support our theories of differences between the sexes.

To explain these stereotypes we must go back to primitive times, when women spent most of their time at home with fellow women and their children. Men, on the other hand, were supposedly out hunting, gathering or fighting. Thus, due to constant communication and social interaction, the emotional part of the female brain developed more effectively – and is now 25 per cent larger, than that of the male.

Scientists have known for a while that men and women have differences in brain structure.

In 2001, researchers at Harvard University found that different parts of the brain were sized differently in men and women. They found that the area responsible for decision – making and problem-solving (the frontal lobe) and the area responsible for regulating emotions (the limbic cortex) were both larger in women. On the other hand, both parts of the brain which regulate sexual and social behaviour (amygdala) and space perception (parietal cortex) were larger in men.

Because of this, women are far better at detecting subtle changes in mood, from facial expressions and tone of voice. Having a more profound emotional brain is also the reason why women tend to spend so much time thinking about their relationships. Men on the other hand, are said to spend more time thinking about sports and work – today's version of hunting and gathering. Whilst this difference in emotional brains is often viewed as a problem, it actually has a useful function in setting the balance in a relationship. The male's emotional tune-out works well in giving protection against distress, so he can stay calm in a crisis while the women's brain focuses on nurture or rescue.

The two brains can work together positively. Thus in a crisis such as a house catching fire, the male might focus on putting the fire out while the female might call for help and rescue the children.

When it comes to recovery from addiction, relationships are often in need of repair. The differences in the emotional brains of men and women can cause problems and misunderstandings. For instance, women may think that their partners are no longer interested in them when they don't talk much during conversations, or when they want to go out with friends instead of staying at home. Men on the other hand, may feel misunderstood because the female partner doesn't recognise their needs for 'space', 'action' or 'challenges'.

Couples working on their relationship might benefit from understanding their brain differences. For example, emotional conversations often stress a man out. Some men can tolerate only a 10-minute emotional conversation. More than this can trigger 'emotional fatigue' and the 'fight or flight' response. When a man starts to show discomfort or seems to be shutting down, some women might turn up the heat at this point, perhaps feeling ignored or rejected but this can result in bigger communication problems; the woman might do better in such a case to keep the conversation short. Luckily, many women are good at sensing emotional discomfort in men even before men realise it themselves (and some men are equally good at this).

Rebuilding a damaged relationship can be one of the biggest challenges in recovery, and understanding a partner's strengths and weaknesses plays a crucial part. The differences between a man and a woman's emotional brain may seem like the source of a problem but they originated for a purpose. They are there not just to create balance, but also to help a couple work together.

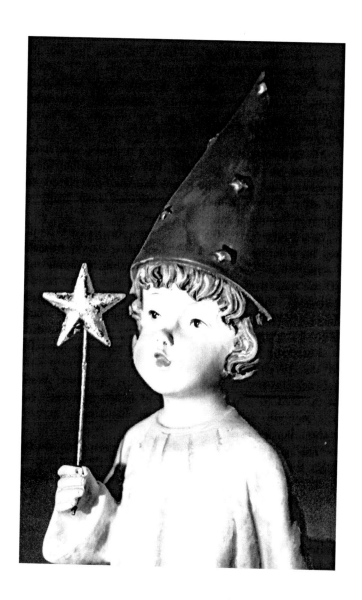

Twelve Triggers of Christmas

Are you 'Dreaming of a White Christmas, just like the ones you used to know'? I'm not: the ones that I used to know were dire – I can best describe them as 'gothic'. Family tensions, overindulgence, selfishness, resentment and bad temper were the norm. The draughty old house felt unwelcoming.

My stepfather would retire with a migraine – he hated Christmas as much as I did. His brooding but silent presence in an upstairs bedroom lent the proceedings the feel of a Victorian novel. Dracula was more likely to appear in the night than Santa Claus.

As a young man, a Christmas visit to my parental family was like entering earth's atmosphere from Mars; it brought a sensation of undefinable terror. Landing on home turf off the train from London I would be very much on the defensive, and this would remain my default mode throughout the festive period. But happily, there would always be enough to drink: I would bring my own supply.

Christmas Eve would be less about expecting the birth of the Messiah as about preventing an all-out fight between me and my siblings. Christmas Day itself would be devoted to false bonhomie and selfish pursuits. That was the only way we could avoid the pain of actually communicating with each other.

This gruesome little scenario was repeated in similar form, for many years. It did not change until I changed.

Today I don't drink but I can still be selfish, judgemental, suspicious, inconsiderate, resentful and generally negative. At Christmas more than at any time, I need to turn this around and become generous, understanding, trusting, loving and generally positive. Believe me, it can still take a big effort. Christmas is an emotional minefield and statistics show that this season of goodwill is also a season of divorce, breakup, breakdown, break the furniture and general mayhem. I cannot afford to buy into the negativity that lurks around the festive tree and nor I suspect, can most recovering addicts or alcoholics. Christmas is also a season of relapse.

Here is my list of twelve triggers – emotions and attitudes to watch at Christmas and some AA thoughts and slogans to help cope with them.

Perhaps you could check yourself for warning signs and take action where needed. Reflect on these items and decide what choices you will make today.

1. Self-pity: Stops real communication – try helping others.

2. Boredom: Work the programme – be pro-active.

3. Pride: For self-acceptance, we need humility.

4. Resentment: How important is it? Help yourself by forgiving.

5. Shame: Let go, let God.

6. Disappointment: Count your blessings.

7. Anxiety: Take it one day at a time. It will pass.

8. Selfishness: Give to others – of yourself.

9. Irresponsibility: Is what you want to do what you need to do?

10. Dishonesty: Total honesty starts with little things.

11. Blaming others: Don't compare – identify.

12. Impatience: King Babies need to grow up.

Too often in the past I have unpacked my angst-filled Christmas stocking of emotions and attitudes, reacting badly, like one of Pavlov's dogs, to each resentment or bad memory that emerges. Changing old patterns of behaviour requires specific effort. I have to remind myself each day that I am an addict and I cannot handle emotions well. I have to do something extra each day to make sure that I don't slip backwards and I have to ask myself each day: is what I want to do today going to keep me emotionally safe? Emotional security depends on vigilance. Doing nothing is not an option, especially at Christmas.

POETRY, PHILOSOPHY AND SPIRITUALITY

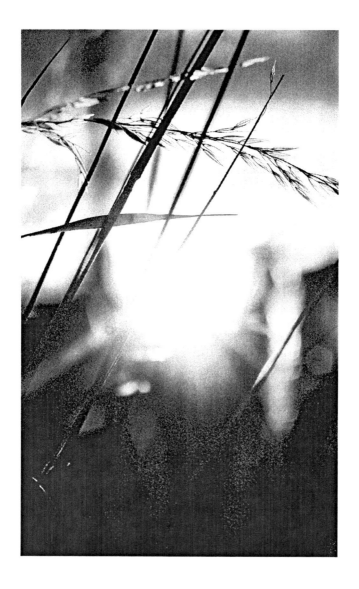

Agnostic Treasure Hunt
An Alternative Serenity Prayer

Jovial Power
Unknown, anonymous,
Laying clues along
The treasure trail of
Acceptance;
Until
I reach
The hidden hoard of
Wisdom.
Hinted presence through
The shimmering leaves of
Hope
Mettles my craven heart.
Companion
Through the labyrinth of
Change –
Into the calm sunshine of
Serenity.

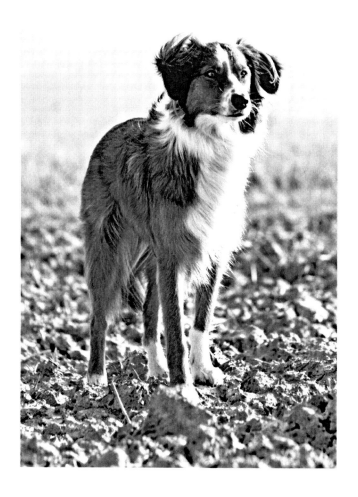

Spirituality and Dogs

A dog provides a different kind of power. Things I have stopped being include, in no particular order of importance: a banker, overweight, a golfer, irresponsible, a problem gambler, self-interested, a practicing alcoholic, and wealthy. Hey Ho, I don't miss any of them. The only other thing I have stopped being is a 'dog owner' and I really do miss my faithful border collie, even after so many years.

Being a dog owner gives you regular exercise, new friends and hairs on your upholstery (none of which you will find around the average banker, but that's enough banker bashing). Being a dog owner also gives you spirituality.

Let me explain. Spirituality provides a meaning to life: it gives an awareness of oneself and a caring regard for others; it takes you out of the centre of the universe and gives you a rightful place amongst equals. I am not surprised to discover that the great majority of those at my local AA meeting – far and away the most spiritual people I know – are dog lovers and most are dog owners. In AA we talk about spirituality a lot. The word 'God' appears a lot too, though we usually say 'Higher Power' because there are many in AA who don't believe in a God of any recognised religion.

For those of us in AA, a Higher Power is what we turn to for help and guidance in recovery from addiction, and it can therefore take many forms. For an atheist it can be his local AA group, for a Christian it can be Jesus Christ, for an agnostic it can simply be a power for good in the world. One thing is for sure though: you want your Higher Power to be the most powerful thing around. Talking about spirituality may seem freaky to some people but discovering their spiritual side is for most people an exciting and life enhancing experience.

So how do dogs come into it? Well, dogs provide a focus of attention outside ourselves; they give unconditional love at all times, they are non-judgemental, honest in displaying their emotions, loyal and forgiving. Pretty handy qualities, I would say.

But can a dog help you in the way that a Higher Power can? Not directly perhaps, and you wouldn't expect to pray to a dog, or to make a dog your higher power (unless you are an ancient Egyptian). To me, a dog provides a different kind of power – the power of example. When I see a dog showing love, feeling happy or being honest, it truly raises my spirits. That power of example has a huge influence on others. Dogs are simpler creatures than us, but they are closer to nature and the power for good that most people believe exists in the world. They are not only man's best friends, but also agents of man's Higher Power.

Many people in the world today have had the spirit drained out of them – life in the 21st century can do that to you. A dog can help to put the spirit back. My daughter Annabel, another big time dog lover, and spiritual down to her socks, has a bumper sticker that runs: "Lord help me to be the person my dog thinks I am". Live up to your dog and you live up to your Higher Power.

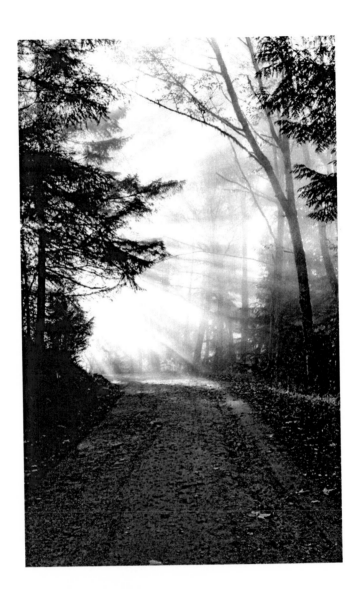

Why the Alchemist is Better than the Chemist

This year I have been enthralled by two stories: first I re-read Paolo Coelho's wonderful book The Alchemist and then later, I watched the TV series Breaking Bad. They could hardly be more different.

Breaking Bad, acclaimed as one of the finest TV series ever written, is the story of Walter White, a struggling high school chemistry teacher who is diagnosed with cancer and decides to provide for his family financially by becoming a crystal-meth producer.

Stating that the end justifies the means, however immoral, he evolves from a caring, compassionate father to a cheating, violent and remorseless murderer over the course of the 62 episodes. He will do anything to get what he wants.

Apart from anything else, it illustrates how unhappy we make ourselves and those around us by ruthlessly pursuing our desires and expectations. Walter White deliberately abandons the light for the darkness.

TV critic Chuck Klosterman says that the central question of Breaking Bad is "what makes a man bad" – his actions, his motives, or his conscious decision to be a bad person?"

The Alchemist, on the other hand, is a beautiful, symbolic and inspirational tale of a boy named Santiago who is on a quest for treasure. He meets an alchemist who shows him that to find his real treasure (i.e. fulfilling his destiny) he must follow his heart.

The book is about the wisdom of listening and learning to read the omens strewn along life's path. These things that Walter White deliberately chooses not to do.

Two very different stories then. But there are similarities. For a start, both Walter and Santiago are on a quest for treasure and both find it, though with very different outcomes: Walter ends up trying to hide tens of millions of drug dollars that he does not live to enjoy, whereas Santiago realises that the gold he can have is unimportant compared to the happiness of fulfilment.

Again, they both have choices to make and they go about making them in very different ways: Walter's choices are made entirely on the basis of doing things his way, so as to achieve the result he wants, no matter what the cost. Santiago's choices are made on the basis of listening to others and to his own heart.

The main theme of The Alchemist is about finding one's destiny. According to The New York Times, The Alchemist is "more self-help than literature". An old king tells Santiago, "when you really want something to happen, the whole universe conspires so that your wish comes true".

This is the book's main philosophy. But, just as in Breaking Bad, Santiago has control over how he wants to live, although here he makes the right choices through seeking guidance.

Towards the end of Breaking Bad Walter tells his horrified wife (to whom he is trying to pass on his ill-gotten treasure), that his behaviour was a deliberate choice and actually he enjoyed all the violence, stealing and murdering because it made him feel alive. In contrast, at the end of The Alchemist, Santiago thinks of the strange way that God had chosen to show him his treasure – he says to himself "the path was written in the omens, and there was no way that I could go wrong".

So what has been the message from these two powerful experiences? I think it is this: as formulas for living go, divine guidance always beats my way. In the end, the Alchemist turned out to be a lot wiser than the Chemist.

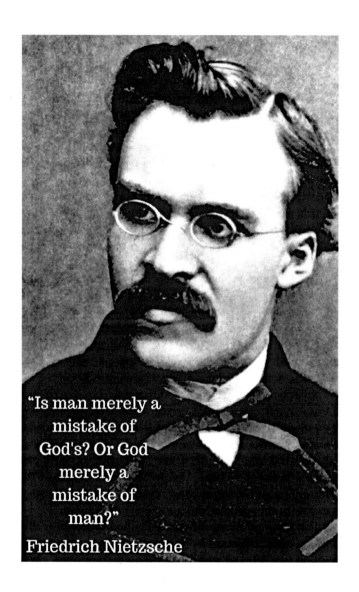

"Is man merely a mistake of God's? Or God merely a mistake of man?"
Friedrich Nietzsche

Is Atheism Better than Religion?

Religious belief is hugely beneficial – physically and psychologically. So says Daily Telegraph writer Sean Thomas in a blog article. A vast body of research, primarily from the US, appears to support this. The University of California published a report which stated that college students involved in religious activities have better mental health than the non-religious students. Meanwhile, researchers at the University of Texas found that the more often you go to church, the longer you live. Harvard's take on the issue is that hospital inmates who are believers have less depression. Other studies show that believers are less likely to commit suicide, cope with stress better and are generally happier than unbelievers. Believers also have more children.

The implication drawn from this is that the human brain is hard-wired for faith and belief, that the species has evolved with an inbuilt religious belief system and that is the reason why believers today are generally happier than unbelievers. Conversely, atheists who lack this vital faculty of faith are seen, by some, as sick people with a tragic affliction akin to blindness; a form of mental illness.

Atheists tend to see things differently. For a start they do not usually agree that believers are the happy ones and they might point to the constant scandals in the Christian church. Plenty of atheists appear to be just as happy as religious folk and probably would agree with the early 20th century political thinker, Annie Besant in saying: 'No philosophy, no religion, has ever brought so glad a message to the world as this good news of Atheism.'

The view of many atheists is rather different – they tend to view religious believers as mentally sick people trapped in a kind of spiritual Stockholm Syndrome , held captive by a God whom they love in spite of the torments and constrictions that he imposes. A far more serious and recognisable condition than theirs, they suggest.

So who is right? Certainly believers obtain support and fellowship through their religions that must increase their sense of wellbeing but no doubt atheists get similar encouragement from scientific evidence and interaction. Perhaps all should ponder the words of that well known atheist, George Bernard Shaw:

"The fact that a believer is happier than a skeptic is no more to the point than the fact that a drunken man is happier than a sober one."

In my view, everyone is entitled to an opinion on such a profound matter without being labelled mentally ill. What I would find really scary would be not having an opinion at all.

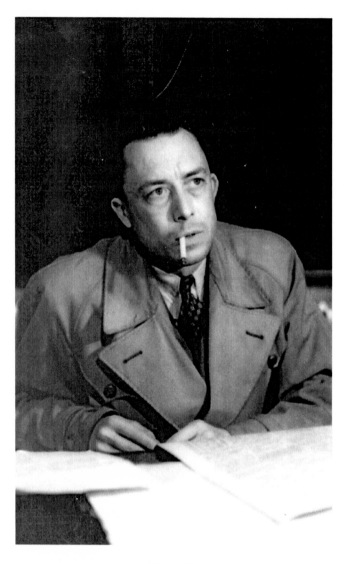

Albert Camus

Pascal's wager?
A good bet, but don't ignore the Outsider

When the great French-Algerian thinker Albert Camus wrote:

'I would rather live my life as if there is a God and die to find out there isn't, than live my life as if there isn't and die to find out there is',

it seemed as if he was echoing the writing of Blaise Pascal three hundred years earlier, who sought to show that belief in God is a rational attitude, with the argument: 'If God does not exist, one will lose nothing by believing in him, while if he does exist, one will lose everything by not believing.' (known later as 'Pascal's wager').

Camus, whose name is always linked to existentialism (though he preferred absurdism) and Pascal, were in fact saying very different things. Both were profound thinkers on the meaning of life, but came to very different conclusions; to Pascal, life is a preparation for the afterlife, to Camus it is an empty absurdity of which we must make the best we can.

Camus, (whose best known work 'The Outsider' (L'Etranger) sets out his own views,) feels that one must live without the pretext of God. Only man is responsible for his life. As existentialist Jean-Paul Sartre put it: 'Man is nothing else but that which he makes of himself.' Therefore when Camus says he would rather live his life as if there is a God, he is only saying that this is a good way to live; he is simply not interested in the question whether God exists or not; to him, it is an irrelevance. As Mersault, the protagonist of 'The Outsider' says, as he lives through his final hours before his public execution: 'I had only a little time left and I didn't want to waste it on God.'

In contrast to this, Pascal, (whose dying words were: 'May God never abandon me'), was a devout Christian whose Pensées are considered a masterpiece which have had a profound effect on religious thinking.

In Pensées, Pascal surveys several philosophical paradoxes such as infinity and oblivion, faith and reason, death and life, concluding that there are no firm answers beyond humility, acceptance and grace in the presence of an all-powerful deity whose existence, he feels, it is reasonable and indeed advisable to assume. Camus deals with similar philosophical issues but comes to radically different conclusions. From a starting point of non-belief ('I have no idea what's awaiting me, or what will happen when this all ends',) he constructs a philosophy based on the premise that the human situation is absurd and unique and it is up to us to take full responsibility for how we live. Far from being a negative view of the world as some suggest, this is an affirmation of human life which, he says, thrives and grows stronger on adversity and suffering:

'In the midst of winter, I found there was, within me, an invincible summer.'

And that makes me happy. For it says that no matter how hard the world pushes against me, within me, there's something stronger – something better, pushing right back.'

Camus sees total honesty without compromise, as the only solution in life. In the Outsider, Mersault could have won leniency if he had been prepared to compromise with the truth (by showing remorse), but he was not. Instead, he found himself, in his final hours, feeling happy and cleansed, as he says:

'For all to be accomplished, for me to feel less lonely, all that remained to hope was that on the day of my execution there should be a huge crowd of spectators and that they should greet me with howls of execration.'

Some commentators have been quick to identify the last days of Mersault – the trial, the refusal to compromise, the public humiliation and death with that of a better known person – yes, Jesus Christ. In writing 'The Outsider', was Camus showing us a glimpse of his real self? He himself said: 'I have tried to portray this character (Mersault) as the only Christ we deserve'. But could it perhaps be that Camus, the man who parodied the words of Christ so grossly when he said 'Right now, all my kingdom is of this world', was having second thoughts?

Actually, stories abound that Camus found God shortly before his tragic death in 1960. There is a certain neatness in this, if it be so. For Camus worshipped Pascal, in spite of their differences in belief, calling him 'Le plus grand de tous, hier et aujourdhui '.

I like to think that Camus in his life made a spiritual journey that took him from meaningless nihilism to the same eventual conclusion as Pascal, who wrote:

'There is a God shaped vacuum in the heart of every man which cannot be filled by any created thing, but only by God, the Creator.'

Perhaps Camus, who once wrote that he had 'devoted his whole life to the attempt to transcend nihilism', succeeded in this quest and finally found a higher power.

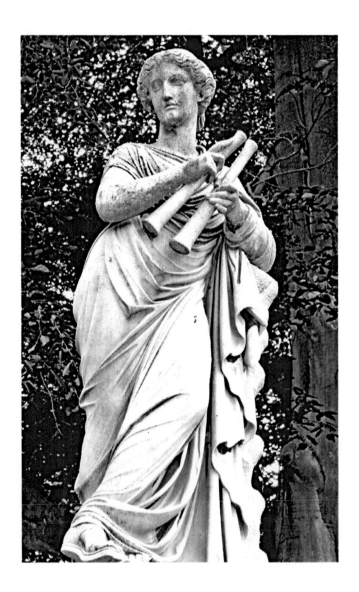

Passion for Poetry:
A Different Kind of Therapy

You're experiencing a bad patch-stress levels high, sleep levels low. You wake every day feeling like roadkill. The world's in a mess, the economy is dire (or at any rate, your economy is dire) – no wonder you feel flattened and empty. In such a state you need some positives: motivation, enthusiasm, inspiration, passion. You need a bit of zing back in your life...

I found my passion in poetry, like many others have since the time when Homer first wrote of 'rosy-fingered dawn lighting the wine-dark sea'. At my lowest ebb, I got a boost from this:

Out of the night that covers me,
Black as the pit from pole to pole,
I thank whatever gods may be,
For my unconquerable soul
(Invictus by W E Henley)

And I was inspired for self-knowledge after reading this:

In me the tiger sniffs the rose.
Look in my heart kind friends and tremble,
Since there your elements assemble.
(Siegfried Sassoon)

My passion gave me back my life and it gave me inspiration. Quite often it was the only thing that got me out of bed in the morning. Poetry puts passion into language and gives words a new interpretation. I love how a poem changes the way we see a familiar event, such as Christmas, 1924, by Thomas Hardy:

'Peace upon earth!' was said. We sing it,
And pay a million priests to bring it.
After two thousand years of mass

We've got as far as poison-gas.

Or the way that poetry draws pictures that aren't really pictures we can see:

The trees are coming into leaf
Like something almost being said
(Philip Larkin)

But most of all I absolutely love the way that poetry makes us feel inside, from AE Houseman's aching nostalgia:

That is the land of lost content,
I see it shining plain.
The happy highways where I went
And cannot come again.

To the unbearable pathos at the ending of Anthem for Doomed Youth by World War I poet Wilfred Owen:

What candles may be held to speed them all?
Not in the hands of boys, but in their eyes
Shall shine the holy glimmers of goodbyes.
The pallor of girls' brows shall be their pall;
Their flowers the tenderness of silent minds,
And each slow dusk a drawing down of blinds.

To EE Cumming's joyously lyrical verses of love from I carry your heart:

I fear no fate (for you are my fate, my sweet)
I want no world (for beautiful you are my world, my true)
and it's you are whatever a moon has always meant
and whatever a sun will always sing is you
here is the deepest secret nobody knows
(here is the root of the root and the bud of the bud and the sky of the sky of a tree called life; which grows higher than the soul can hope or mind can hide)
and this is the wonder that's keeping the stars apart

I carry your heart (I carry it in my heart).

To the quiet contentment of Raymond Carver's dying thoughts in Late Frangment:

And did you get what
You wanted from this life, even so?
I did.
And what did you want?
To call myself beloved,
To feel myself beloved,
On the earth.

Is any of this getting through to you? It is to me, I'm starting to get quite emotional. Time for a comfort break.

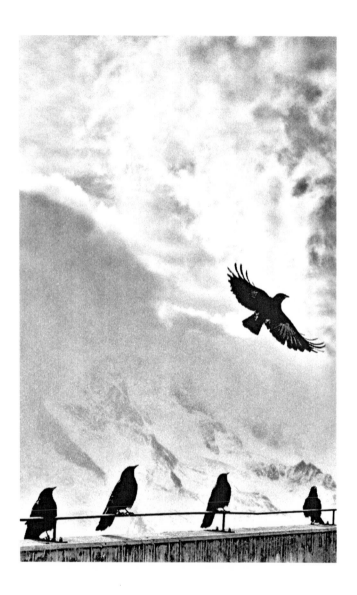

Make Poetry

You don't like reading poetry? Try writing it then. Modern poetry can be fun. Try the 'cut-up' poetry technique used by American writer and lifelong heroin junkie William Burroughs, where printed material is cut up and assembled at random. Here's one I made earlier:

The book you have in your hands,
Confers the most benefits,
Dancing, singing and drinking,
By which we are able to bear
What comes to pass.
I used your product and have never looked back.

Or try writing a Haiku (a three-line Japanese poem of seventeen syllables) – just aim to express what's in your head. Here is one:

Summer's nearly here.
The swallows are returning.
All life is renewed.

That took me all of two minutes to write and can certainly be improved, but I enjoyed it. If nothing else, poetry helps you to express your feelings, something many of us do not find easy. It can help with any feeling, even boredom.

I composed this while driving slowly in heavy traffic up the A9 road, North of Inverness:

Across the road and far afield
The golden landscape shines,
Although the local wind farm blocks
The view of power lines.
From all around a whooshing sound
Comes bouncing off the hills,
For far and wide the countryside
Is white satanic mills.

It's actually very easy to write poetry, though writing good poetry is something else; but that will come, with time, one hopes (some of us have been waiting a long time). Poetry doesn't have to rhyme, though rhyming can really help to keep a rhythm going. Poets like TS Eliot often use rhyme on an occasional basis to give emphasis to a word picture such as:

> The nightingales are singing near
> The convent of the Sacred Heart,
> And sang within the bloody wood
> Where Agamemnon cried aloud,
> And let their liquid siftings fall
> To stain the stiff dishonoured shroud.

Modern poetry is often a narrative of banal experience expressed in a special way. I like this one by American poet Jack Gilbert – try telling a simple experience yourself:

> Quietly, I look in the bus waiting
> Next to us and meet the eyes
> Of a pretty Greek girl.
> She looks back steadily.
> I drop my eyes and the bus
> Drives away.

The main point is that poetry can be easy and enjoyable to write; even when the lines themselves are not immortal, the act of writing can give the writer great pleasure. Who knows, one day it might even give the reader pleasure too. Poetry changes lives – it really does, and the Poetry gives life to otherwise stodgy facts. It can make you creative, busy, focused and positive. It can actually make you happy too. Poetry inspires, soothes and delights. It can become an absorbing interest and more. It is my passion and my delight and it took me on a journey from being nothing to being something.

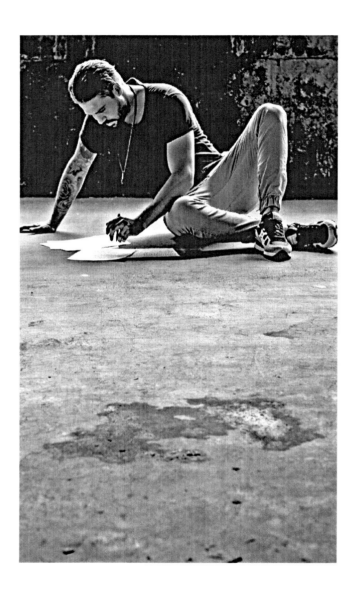

Poetry as Therapy

What did Abraham Lincoln, Albert Einstein, Pope John Paul II and Marilyn Monroe have in common? As you may have guessed, they all wrote poetry. The question one could ask is – why? All of them were highly successful in their chosen careers which were demanding, stressful and far removed from literature. Did they see writing poetry as a therapy? Perhaps a relaxation, a means of expressing their true feelings, a way of coping with life's difficulties, a way of defining who they really were, or what? All the above mentioned experienced great personal stress during their lives.

Can people use poetry to help them in such times of crisis? The ancient Greeks and Romans certainly believed that: "words are the physician of the mind diseased." and Apollo was the god of both healing and the arts.

A lot of poetry was written by the condemned on the eve of their execution – Sir Thomas More is an example. Here is the very last thing he wrote – To Fortune – a little poem written using a piece of coal in his cell, on the night before he was beheaded:

But in faith I bless you again a thousand times,

For lending me now some leisure to make rhymes

Not perhaps great poetry but interesting in that he felt the need to express himself thus at such a terrible moment.

The fact is that people do turn to poetry in times of trauma and great emotional upheaval; history is full of examples of this from Homer's Troy to the World War I poets. After 9/11 thousands of poems were written and posted at the site. After the school shootings at Columbine, eyewitnesses and others closely affected were encouraged to use poetry to begin the healing process.

Poetry has been around since recorded history began and in fact was the earliest way of recording history. The earliest poem ever found was written on a Sumerian clay tablet about 2000BC. It was discovered in a region that is now part of Iraq in the 1880s. It is now in the Istanbul Museum of the Ancient Orient. Here is an extract:

Bridegroom, dear to my heart,
Goodly is your beauty, honeysweet.
You have captivated me,
Let me stand trembling before you;
I would be taken to your bedchamber.

This is clearly an expression of feelings just as real as Sylvia Plath's words 4000 years later:

The stars go waltzing out in blue and red,
And arbitrary blackness gallops in:
I shut my eyes and all the world drops dead.
I dreamed that you bewitched me into bed
And sung me moon-struck, kissed me quite insane.
(I think I made you up inside my head.)

Both these poems have great power for enjoyment. But both examples, were probably written not just to give pleasure, but also to help the writer deal with their own emotions – a kind of therapy; If nothing else, poetry is the voice of the soul. And when the soul is in torment, even for the sweet agony of love, it cries out for expression. Overpowering feelings such as grief or, in this case, love, need to be expressed and writing poetry is the self-medication, the therapy that is always available, just as it was four thousand years ago.

Here is another example. This poem by Billy Collins shows how the writer changes his own attitude and manages to turn a difficult situation into a joke. In other words, he uses the act of writing the poem to change the way he feels:

The neighbors' dog will not stop barking.
He is barking the same high, rhythmic bark
that he barks every time they leave the house.
They must switch him on on their way out.

The neighbors' dog will not stop barking.
I close all the windows in the house
and put on a Beethoven symphony full blast...

...When the record finally ends he is still barking,
sitting there in the oboe section barking,
his eyes fixed on the conductor who is
entreating him with his baton
while the other musicians listen in respectful
silence to the famous barking dog solo,
that endless coda that first established
Beethoven as an innovative genius.
(part of Another Reason Why I Don't Keep a Gun in
the House by Billy Collins)

A poem that can make a chronically barking dog seem funny has got to be powerful therapy. It shows us that poetry can change the way we feel. The act of reading or writing poetry can either bring us an acceptance of our situation or it can be a catalyst for change. And acceptance and change are the basic processes of therapy.

Some practitioners in the field are coming to realise the importance of poetry as therapy:

'I now think poetry has more capacity to change people than psychotherapy. If you read a poem and it gets to you, it can shift your perspective in quite a big way, and writing a poem, even more so.' (Sean Haldane, poet and consultant clinical neuropsychologist, nominee for the post of professor of poetry at Oxford University.)

The power of poetry to calm, to inspire, to express feelings and to change them, and ultimately to heal, should not be underestimated. In our troubled world we need all the help that we can get.

Writing, reading or visualising poetry are methods being used increasingly in therapy, particularly in trauma and bereavement cases. In Europe this is less common than in the United States, where The National Federation for Poetry Therapy (www.poetrytherapy.org), incorporated in 1963, sets standards of excellence in the training and qualifying of practitioners.

Well known practitioners and authors of books on poetry therapy include Nicholas Mazza and John Fox in the USA and Diana Hedges and Geri Giebel Chavis in the UK.

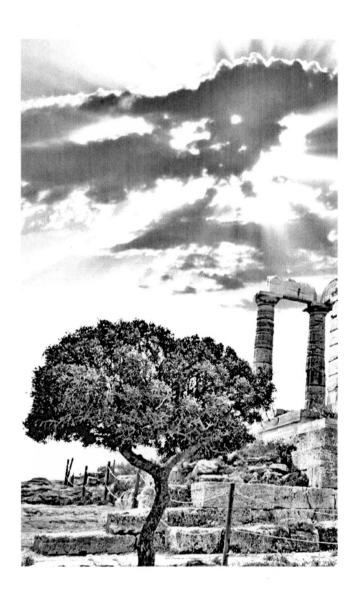

Unknown God

In ancient Athens there was a famous shrine 'to an Unknown God' (Ἄγνωστος Θεός). St Paul saw this when he visited Athens in AD 51 and he proceeded to berate the Athenians for their (as he saw it) ignorance and sloppy religious attitude. It gave rise to one of his most famous sermons in which he set out to define the meaning of his Christian God, whose word he was preaching with all the zeal of his recent conversion.

Many people now, take the opposite view to Paul, (as many did then): the Athenians were not ignorant and sloppy – their idea of deity and religion was in fact direct and existential, based on respect and personal responsibility: live your life as best you can and ask for help when you need it. The idea of original sin, guilt and redemption would have been quite alien. Hardly surprising then that, according to St Luke, many Athenians laughed at Paul's sermon. The ancient Greek religion was simple, eclectic and mostly non-evangelical; in fact very relaxed and civilised.

On the other hand, the great philosopher Friedrich Nietzsche had this to say about Christianity – he makes it sound more like torture than divine guidance:

'The Christian faith is from the beginning sacrifice: sacrifice of all freedom, all pride, all self-confidence of the spirit, at the same time self-mockery, self-mutilation.'

The Athenians in AD51 had barely heard the word 'Christianity' let alone 'Nietzsche' (lucky them), but they knew what they wanted – how to deal with life, and their philosophies of Stoicism, Epicureanism and the like were designed for this purpose. Deeds in other words, not dogma.

The Ancient Greeks often remind me of AA. Their grasp of the essential truths; their refusal to compromise; and of course the Delphic Oracle with its famous slogans 'water is best', 'nothing in excess' and 'know thyself'.

When they dedicated a shrine to an Unknown God, they were in effect acknowledging the existence of a Higher Power in their lives which defied exact definition through its very nature. They were happy to accept the reality of the power without feeling the need to cloak it in religion. The power, in other words, was the important thing, not the religion. One can imagine them shouting out the AA slogans to Paul – 'keep it simple', 'first things first', 'how important is it?'

A lot of recovering addicts have this 'Unknown God' – they call it 'A Power Greater than Themselves' and it serves them well, as it did the Athenians.

The truth is that nobody knows God in an empirical sense. How can we possibly? Just a look at our corner of the Universe should tell us that it is beyond belief. Billions of light years separate us from some galaxies but we can't even be sure that our concept of distance, time and space is right. It is as they say, beyond belief. It all puts me in mind of that mysterious poem of Ralph Waldo Emerson :

Far or forgot to me is near;
Shadow and sunlight are the same;
The vanished gods to me appear;
And one to me are shame and fame.
They reckon ill who leave me out;
When me they fly, I am the wings;
I am the doubter and the doubt,
And I the hymn the Brahmin sings

Very few things for me have been a consistent power for good over the entire course of my lifetime. AA is certainly one, perhaps the only shining example that I know, whereas the various world religions, sadly, have not been so.

Someone once said that, considering all the religious sects and beliefs there are, that they hoped God had a sense of humour. I hope so too. I wish more people did as well. Particularly religious ones. Exploring spirituality is fascinating, exciting and even amusing at times; exploring religion these days, is not.

ABOUT THE AUTHOR

Christopher Burn is a writer and psychotherapist. He is also a Chartered Accountant, recovering alcoholic, father of three and grandfather of five. He is interested in poetry, history, spirituality and the universe, in no particular order of priority. Christopher divides his time between Scotland and London.

Christopher also published Poetry Changes Lives, a book of daily meditations drawing inspiration from poetry and history (available as paperback or ebook).

To find out more and get in touch with the author, visit: www.poetrychangeslives.com.

Lightning Source UK Ltd.
Milton Keynes UK
UKOW02f1549051116
286879UK00001B/23/P